My Favorite Air Fryer Recipes

Quick and Refreshing Smoothies to Enjoy Your Diet and Boost Your Metabolism

Dalia Gillespie

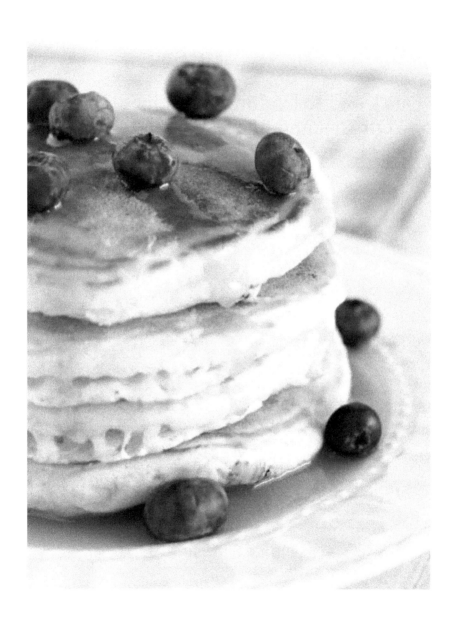

this book has been derived from various sources. Please consult a licensed professional before attempting any techniques outlined in this book.

By reading this document, the reader agrees that under no circumstances is the author responsible for any losses, direct or indirect, which are incurred as a result of the use of information contained within this document, including, but not limited to, — errors, omissions, or inaccuracies.

TABLE OF CONTENT

White Chocolate Chip Cookies

Preparation Time: 30 min

Servings: 8

Nutrition Values: Calories: 167; Carbs: 21.3g; Fat: 11.3g; Protein: 0.7g

Ingredients

- 6 oz self-rising flour
- 3 oz brown sugar
- 2 oz white chocolate chips
- 1 tbsp honey
- 1 ½ tbsp milk
- 4 oz butter

Directions

1. Preheat the Air fryer to 350 F, and beat the butter and sugar until fluffy. Beat in the honey, milk, and flour. Gently fold in the chocolate chips. Drop spoonfuls of the mixture onto a prepared cookie sheet. Cook for 18 minutes.

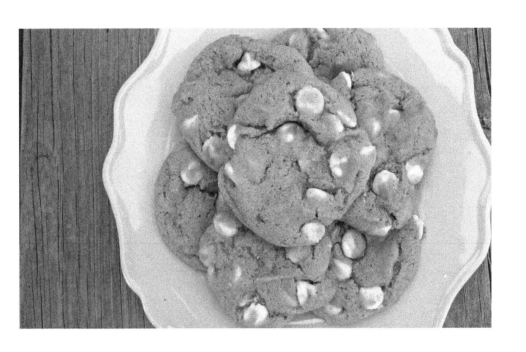

White Filling Coconut and Oat Cookies

Preparation Time: 30 min

Servings: 4

Nutrition Values: Calories: 477; Carbs: 73.8g; Fat: 16.8g; Protein: 7.4g

Ingredients

- 5 ½ oz flour
- 1 tsp vanilla extract
- 3 oz sugar
- ½ cup oats
- 1 small egg, beaten
- ¼ cup coconut flakes

Filling:

- 1 oz white chocolate, melted
- 2 oz butter
- 4 oz powdered sugar
- 1 tsp vanilla extract

Directions

1. Beat all the cookie ingredients, with an electric mixer, except the flour. When

smooth, fold in the flour. Drop spoonfuls of the batter onto a prepared cookie sheet. Cook in the Air fryer at 350 F for 18 minutes; then let cool.

2. Meanwhile, prepare the filling by beating all ingredients together; spread the filling on half of the cookies. Top with the other halves to make cookie sandwiches.

Tasty Banana Cake

Preparation time: 10 minutes

Cooking time: 30 minutes

Servings: 4

Ingredients:

- 1 tablespoon butter, soft
- 1 egg
- 1/3 cup brown sugar
- 2 tablespoons honey
- 1 banana, peeled and mashed
- 1 cup white flour
- 1 teaspoon baking powder
- ½ teaspoon cinnamon powder
- Cooking spray

Directions:

1. Spray a cake pan with some cooking spray and leave aside.

2. In a bowl, mix butter with sugar, banana, honey, egg, cinnamon, baking powder and flour and whisk

3. Pour this into a cake pan greased with cooking spray, introduce in your air fryer and cook at 350 degrees F for 30 minutes.

4. Leave cake to cool down, slice and serve.

5. Enjoy!

Nutrition Values: calories 232, fat 4, fiber 1, carbs 34, protein 4

Simple Cheesecake

Preparation time: 10 minutes

Cooking time: 15 minutes

Servings: 15

Ingredients:

- 1 pound cream cheese
- ½ teaspoon vanilla extract
- 2 eggs
- 4 tablespoons sugar
- 1 cup graham crackers, crumbled
- 2 tablespoons butter

Directions:

1. In a bowl, mix crackers with butter.

2. Press crackers mix on the bottom of a lined cake pan, introduce in your air fryer and cook at 350 degrees F for 4 minutes.

3. Meanwhile, in a bowl, mix sugar with cream cheese, eggs and vanilla and whisk well.

4. Spread filling over crackers crust and cook your cheesecake in your air fryer at 310 degrees F for 15 minutes.

5. Leave cake in the fridge for 3 hours, slice and serve.

6. Enjoy!

Nutrition Values: calories 245, fat 12, fiber 1, carbs 20, protein 3

Bread Pudding

Preparation time: 10 minutes

Cooking time: 1 hour

Servings: 4

Ingredients:

- 6 glazed doughnuts, crumbled
- 1 cup cherries
- 4 egg yolks
- 1 and ½ cups whipping cream
- ½ cup raisins
- ¼ cup sugar
- ½ cup chocolate chips.

Directions:

1. In a bowl, mix cherries with egg yolks and whipping cream and stir well.

2. In another bowl, mix raisins with sugar, chocolate chips and doughnuts and stir.

3. Combine the 2 mixtures, transfer everything to a greased pan that fits your air fryer and cook at 310 degrees F for 1 hour.

4. Chill pudding before cutting and serving it.

5. Enjoy!

Nutrition Values: calories 302, fat 8, fiber 2, carbs 23, protein 10

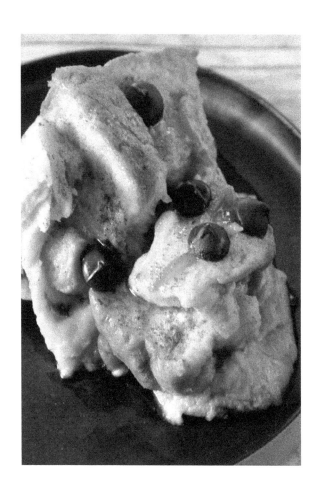

Bread Dough and Amaretto Dessert

Preparation time: 10 minutes

Cooking time: 12 minutes

Servings: 12

Ingredients:

- 1 pound bread dough
- 1 cup sugar
- ½ cup butter, melted
- 1 cup heavy cream
- 12 ounces chocolate chips
- 2 tablespoons amaretto liqueur

Directions:

1. Roll dough, cut into 20 slices and then cut each slice in halves.

2. Brush dough pieces with butter, sprinkle sugar, place them in your air fryer's basket after you've brushed it some butter, cook them at 350 degrees F for 5 minutes, flip them, cook for 3 minutes more and transfer to a platter.

3. Heat up a pan with the heavy cream over medium heat, add chocolate chips and stir until they melt.

4. Add liqueur, stir again, transfer to a bowl and serve bread dippers with this sauce.

5. Enjoy!

Nutrition Values: calories 200, fat 1, fiber 0, carbs 6, protein 6

Cinnamon Rolls and Cream Cheese Dip

Preparation time: 2 hours

Cooking time: 15 minutes

Servings: 8

Ingredients:

- 1 pound bread dough
- ¾ cup brown sugar
- 1 and ½ tablespoons cinnamon, ground
- ¼ cup butter, melted
- For the cream cheese dip:
- 2 tablespoons butter
- 4 ounces cream cheese
- 1 and ¼ cups sugar
- ½ teaspoon vanilla

Directions:

1. Roll dough on a floured working surface, shape a rectangle and brush with ¼ cup butter.

2. In a bowl, mix cinnamon with sugar, stir, sprinkle this over dough, roll dough into a log, seal well and cut into 8 pieces.

3. Leave rolls to rise for 2 hours, place them in your air fryer's basket, cook at 350 degrees F for 5 minutes, flip them, cook for 4 minutes more and transfer to a platter.

4. In a bowl, mix cream cheese with butter, sugar and vanilla and whisk really well.

5. Serve your cinnamon rolls with this cream cheese dip.

6. Enjoy!

Nutrition Values: calories 200, fat 1, fiber 0, carbs 5, protein 6

Pumpkin Pie

Preparation time: 10 minutes

Cooking time: 15 minutes

Servings: 9

Ingredients:

- 1 tablespoon sugar
- 2 tablespoons flour
- 1 tablespoon butter
- 2 tablespoons water

For the pumpkin pie filling:

- ounces pumpkin flesh, chopped
- 1 teaspoon mixed spice
- 1 teaspoon nutmeg
- 3 ounces water
- 1 egg, whisked
- 1 tablespoon sugar

Directions:

1. Put 3 ounces water in a pot, bring to a boil over medium high heat, add pumpkin, egg, 1 tablespoon sugar, spice and nutmeg, stir,

boil for 20 minutes, take off heat and blend using an immersion blender.

2. In a bowl, mix flour with butter, 1 tablespoon sugar and 2 tablespoons water and knead your dough well.

3. Grease a pie pan that fits your air fryer with butter, press dough into the pan, fill with pumpkin pie filling, place in your air fryer's basket and cook at 360 degrees F for 15 minutes.

4. Slice and serve warm.

5. Enjoy!

Nutrition Values: calories 200, fat 5, fiber 2, carbs 5, protein 6

Wrapped Pears

Preparation time: 10 minutes

Cooking time: 15 minutes

Servings: 4

Ingredients:

- 4 puff pastry sheets
- 14 ounces vanilla custard
- 2 pears, halved
- 1 egg, whisked
- ½ teaspoon cinnamon powder
- 2 tablespoons sugar

Directions:

1. Place puff pastry slices on a working surface, add spoonfuls of vanilla custard in the center of each, top with pear halves and wrap.

2. Brush pears with egg, sprinkle sugar and cinnamon, place them in your air fryer's basket and cook at 320 degrees F for 15 minutes.

3. Divide parcels on plates and serve.

4. Enjoy!

Nutrition Values: calories 200, fat 2, fiber 1, carbs 14, protein 3

Strawberry Donuts

Preparation time: 10 minutes

Cooking time: 15 minutes

Servings: 4

Ingredients:

- 8 ounces flour
- 1 tablespoon brown sugar
- 1 tablespoon white sugar
- 1 egg
- 2 and ½ tablespoons butter
- 4 ounces whole milk
- 1 teaspoon baking powder
- For the strawberry icing:
- 2 tablespoons butter
- ounces icing sugar
- ½ teaspoon pink coloring
- ¼ cup strawberries, chopped
- 1 tablespoon whipped cream

Directions:

1. In a bowl, mix butter, 1 tablespoon brown sugar, 1 tablespoon white sugar and flour and stir.

2. In a second bowl, mix egg with 1 and ½ tablespoons butter and milk and stir well.

3. Combine the 2 mixtures, stir, shape donuts from this mix, place them in your air fryer's basket and cook at 360 degrees F for 15 minutes.

4. Put 1 tablespoon butter, icing sugar, food coloring, whipped cream and strawberry puree and whisk well.

5. Arrange donuts on a platter and serve with strawberry icing on top.

6. Enjoy!

Nutrition Values: calories 250, fat 12, fiber 1, carbs 32, protein 4

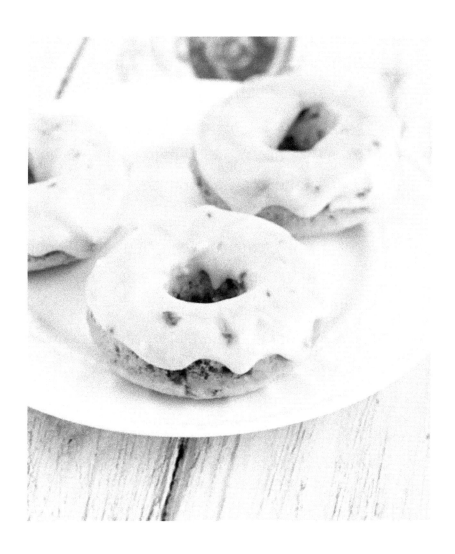

Air Fried Bananas

Preparation time: 10 minutes

Cooking time: 15 minutes

Servings: 4

Ingredients:

- 3 tablespoons butter
- 2 eggs
- 8 bananas, peeled and halved
- ½ cup corn flour
- 3 tablespoons cinnamon sugar
- 1 cup panko

Directions:

1. Heat up a pan with the butter over medium high heat, add panko, stir and cook for 4 minutes and then transfer to a bowl.

2. Roll each in flour, eggs and panko mix, arrange them in your air fryer's basket, dust with cinnamon sugar and cook at 280 degrees F for 10 minutes.

3. Serve right away.

4. Enjoy!

Nutrition Values: calories 164, fat 1, fiber 4, carbs 32, protein 4

Cocoa Cake

Preparation time: 10 minutes

Cooking time: 17 minutes

Servings: 6

Ingredients:

- ounces butter, melted
- 3 eggs
- 3 ounces sugar
- 1 teaspoon cocoa powder
- 3 ounces flour
- ½ teaspoon lemon juice

Directions:

1. In a bowl, mix 1 tablespoon butter with cocoa powder and whisk.

2. In another bowl, mix the rest of the butter with sugar, eggs, flour and lemon juice, whisk well and pour half into a cake pan that fits your air fryer.

3. Add half of the cocoa mix, spread, add the rest of the butter layer and top with the rest of cocoa.

4. Introduce in your air fryer and cook at 360 degrees F for 17 minutes.

5. Cool cake down before slicing and serving.

6. Enjoy!

Nutrition Values: calories 340, fat 11, fiber 3, carbs 25, protein 5

Chocolate Cake

Preparation time: 10 minutes

Cooking time: 30 minutes

Servings: 12

Ingredients:

- ¾ cup white flour
- ¾ cup whole wheat flour
- 1 teaspoon baking soda
- ¾ teaspoon pumpkin pie spice
- ¾ cup sugar
- 1 banana, mashed
- ½ teaspoon baking powder
- 2 tablespoons canola oil
- ½ cup Greek yogurt
- 8 ounces canned pumpkin puree
- Cooking spray
- 1 egg
- ½ teaspoon vanilla extract
- 2/3 cup chocolate chips

Directions:

1. In a bowl, mix white flour with whole wheat flour, salt, baking soda and powder and pumpkin spice and stir.

2. In another bowl, mix sugar with oil, banana, yogurt, pumpkin puree, vanilla and egg and stir using a mixer.

3. Combine the 2 mixtures, add chocolate chips, stir, pour this into a greased Bundt pan that fits your air fryer.

4. Introduce in your air fryer and cook at 330 degrees F for 30 minutes.

5. Leave the cake to cool down, before cutting and serving it.

6. Enjoy!

Nutrition Values: calories 232, fat 7, fiber 7, carbs 29, protein 4

Apple Bread

Preparation time: 10 minutes

Cooking time: 40 minutes

Servings: 6

Ingredients:

- 3 cups apples, cored and cubed
- 1 cup sugar
- 1 tablespoon vanilla
- 2 eggs
- 1 tablespoon apple pie spice
- 2 cups white flour
- 1 tablespoon baking powder
- 1 stick butter
- 1 cup water

Directions:

1. In a bowl mix egg with 1 butter stick, apple pie spice and sugar and stir using your mixer.

2. Add apples and stir again well.

3. In another bowl, mix baking powder with flour and stir.

4. Combine the 2 mixtures, stir and pour into a spring form pan.

5. Put spring form pan in your air fryer and cook at 320 degrees F for 40 minutes

6. Slice and serve.

7. Enjoy!

Nutrition Values: calories 192, fat 6, fiber 7, carbs 14, protein 7

Banana Bread

Preparation time: 10 minutes

Cooking time: 40 minutes

Servings: 6

Ingredients:

- ¾ cup sugar
- 1/3 cup butter
- 1 teaspoon vanilla extract
- 1 egg
- 2 bananas, mashed
- 1 teaspoon baking powder
- 1 and ½ cups flour
- ½ teaspoons baking soda
- 1/3 cup milk
- 1 and ½ teaspoons cream of tartar
- Cooking spray

Directions:

1. In a bowl, mix milk with cream of tartar, sugar, butter, egg, vanilla and bananas and stir everything.

2. In another bowl, mix flour with baking powder and baking soda.

3. Combine the 2 mixtures, stir well, pour this into a cake pan greased with some cooking spray, introduce in your air fryer and cook at 320 degrees F for 40 minutes.

4. Take bread out, leave aside to cool down, slice and serve it.

5. Enjoy!

Nutrition Values: calories 292, fat 7, fiber 8, carbs 28, protein 4

Mini Lava Cakes

Preparation time: 10 minutes

Cooking time: 20 minutes

Servings: 3

Ingredients:

- 1 egg
- 4 tablespoons sugar
- 2 tablespoons olive oil
- 4 tablespoons milk
- 4 tablespoons flour
- 1 tablespoon cocoa powder
- ½ teaspoon baking powder
- ½ teaspoon orange zest

Directions:

1. In a bowl, mix egg with sugar, oil, milk, flour, salt, cocoa powder, baking powder and orange zest, stir very well and pour this into greased ramekins.

2. Add ramekins to your air fryer and cook at 320 degrees F for 20 minutes.

3. Serve lava cakes warm.

4. Enjoy!

Nutrition Values: calories 201, fat 7, fiber 8, carbs 23, protein 4

Mini Strawberry Pies with Sugar Crust

Preparation Time: 15 minutes

Servings 8

Nutrition Values:237 Calories; 12.8g Fat; 28.2g Carbs; 2.7g Protein; 8.9g Sugars

Ingredients

- 1/2 cup powdered sugar
- 1/4 teaspoon ground cloves
- 1/8 teaspoon cinnamon powder
- 1 teaspoon vanilla extract
- 1 -12-ouncecan biscuit dough
- 12 ounces strawberry pie filling
- 1/4 cup butter, melted

Directions

1. Thoroughly combine the sugar, cloves, cinnamon, and vanilla.

2. Then, stretch and flatten each piece of the biscuit dough into a round circle using a rolling pin.

3. Divide the strawberry pie filling among the biscuits. Roll up tightly and dip each biscuit piece into the melted butter; cover them with the spiced sugar mixture.

4. Brush with a non-stick cooking oil on all sides. Air-bake them at 340 degrees F for approximately 10 minutes or until they're golden brown. Let them cool for 5 minutes before serving.

Fudgy Coconut Brownies

Preparation Time: 15 minutes

Servings 8

Nutrition Values:267 Calories; 15.4g Fat; 34.0g Carbs; 1.0g Protein; 27.5g Sugars

Ingredients

- 1/2 cup coconut oil
- 2 ounces dark chocolate
- 1 cup sugar
- 2 ½ tablespoons water
- 4 whisked eggs
- 1/4 teaspoon ground cinnamon
- 1/2 teaspoon ground anise star
- 1/4 teaspoon coconut extract
- 1/2 teaspoon vanilla extract
- 1 tablespoon honey
- 1/2 cup cake flour
- 1/2 cup desiccated coconut
- Icing sugar, to dust

Directions

1. Microwave the coconut oil along with dark chocolate. Stir in sugar, water, eggs, cinnamon, anise, coconut extract, vanilla, and honey.

2. After that, stir in the flour and coconut; mix to combine thoroughly.

3. Press the mixture into a lightly buttered baking dish. Air-bake at 355 degrees F for 15 minutes.

4. Let your brownie cool slightly; then, carefully remove from the baking dish and cut into squares. Dust with icing sugar. Bon appétit!

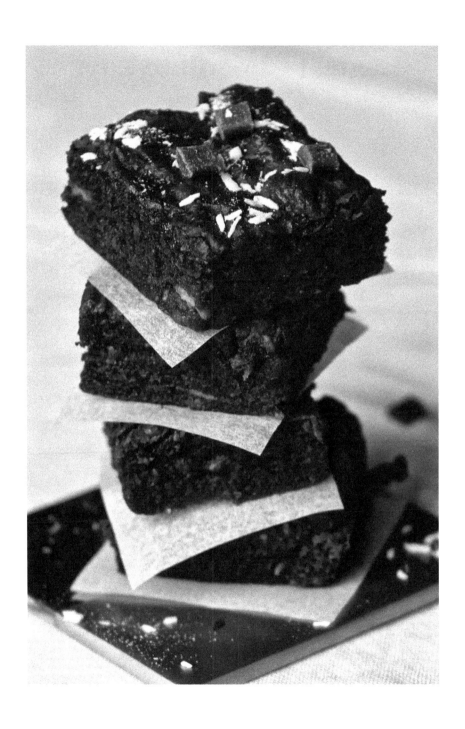

Easiest Chocolate Lava Cake Ever

Preparation Time: 20 minutes

Servings 4

Nutrition Values:549 Calories; 37.7g Fat; 47.5g Carbs; 7.1g Protein; 38.2g Sugars

Ingredients

- 1 cup dark cocoa candy melts
- 1 stick butter
- 2 eggs
- 4 tablespoons superfine sugar
- 1 tablespoon honey
- 4 tablespoons self-rising flour
- A pinch of kosher salt
- A pinch of ground cloves
- 1/4 teaspoon grated nutmeg
- 1/4 teaspoon cinnamon powder

Directions

1. Firstly, spray four custard cups with non-stick cooking oil.

2. Put the cocoa candy melts and butter into a small microwave-safe bowl; microwave on high for 30 seconds to 1 minute.

3. In a mixing bowl, whisk the eggs along with sugar and honey until frothy. Add it to the chocolate mix.

4. After that, add the remaining ingredients and mix to combine well. You can whisk the mixture with an electric mixer.

5. Spoon the mixture into the prepared custard cups. Air-bake at 350 degrees F for 12 minutes. Take the cups out of the Air Fryer and let them rest for 5 to 6 minutes.

6. Lastly, flip each cup upside-down onto a dessert plate and serve with some fruits and chocolate syrup. Bon appétit!

Chocolate Banana Cake

Preparation Time: 30 minutes

Servings 10

Nutrition Values:263 Calories; 10.6g Fat; 41.0g Carbs; 4.3g Protein; 16.6g Sugars

Ingredients

- 1 stick softened butter
- 1/2 cup caster sugar
- 1 egg
- 2 bananas, mashed
- 3 tablespoons maple syrup
- 2 cups self-rising flour
- 1/4 teaspoon anise star, ground
- 1/4 teaspoon ground mace
- 1/4 teaspoon ground cinnamon
- 1/4 teaspoon crystallized ginger
- 1/2 teaspoon vanilla paste
- A pinch of kosher salt
- 1/2 cup cocoa powder

Directions

1. Firstly, beat the softened butter and sugar until well combined.

2. Then, whisk the egg, mashed banana and maple syrup. Now, add this mixture to the butter mixture; mix until pale and creamy.

3. Add in the flour, anise star, mace, cinnamon, crystallized ginger, vanilla paste, and the salt; now, add the cocoa powder and mix to combine.

4. Then, treat two cake pans with a non-stick cooking spray. Press the batter into the cake pans.

5. Air-bake at 330 degrees F for 30 minutes. To serve, frost with chocolate butter glaze.

Butter Sugar Fritters

Preparation Time: 30 minutes

Servings 16

Nutrition Values:231 Calories; 8.2g Fat; 36.6g
Carbs; 3.3g Protein; 12.8g Sugars

Ingredients

For the dough:

- 4 cups fine cake flour
- 1 teaspoon kosher salt
- 1 teaspoon brown sugar
- 3 tablespoons butter, at room temperature
- 1 packet instant yeast
- 1 ¼ cups lukewarm water

For the Cakes:

- 1 cup caster sugar
- A pinch of cardamom
- 1 teaspoon cinnamon powder
- 1 stick butter, melted

Directions

1. Mix all the dry ingredients in a large-sized bowl; add the butter and yeast and mix to combine well.

2. Pour lukewarm water and stir to form soft and elastic dough.

3. Lay the dough on a lightly floured surface, loosely cover with greased foil and chill for 5 to 10 minutes.

4. Take the dough out of the refrigerator and shape it into two logs; cut them into 20 slices.

5. In a shallow bowl, mix caster sugar with cardamom and cinnamon.

6. Now, brush with melted butter and coat the entire slice with sugar mix; repeat with the remaining ingredients.

7. Treat the Air Fryer basket with a non-stick cooking spray. Air-fry at 360 degrees F for about 10 minutes, flipping once during the baking time. To serve, dust with icing sugar and enjoy!

Father's Day Fried Pineapple Rings

Preparation Time: 10 minutes

Servings 6

Nutrition Values:180 Calories; 1.8g Fat; 39.4g Carbs; 2.5g Protein; 14.9g Sugars

Ingredients

- 2/3 cup all-purpose flour
- 1/3 cup rice flour
- 1/2 teaspoon baking powder
- 1/2 teaspoon baking soda
- A pinch of kosher salt
- 1/2 cup water
- 1 cup rice milk
- 1/2 teaspoon ground cinnamon
- 1/4 teaspoon ground anise star
- 1/2 teaspoon vanilla essence
- 4 tablespoons caster sugar
- 1/4 cup unsweetened flaked coconut
- 1 medium-sized pineapple, peeled and sliced

Directions

1. Mix all of the above ingredients, except the pineapple. Then, coat the pineapple slices with the batter mix, covering well.

2. Air-fry them at 380 degrees F for 6 to 8 minutes. Drizzle with maple syrup, garnish with a dollop of vanilla ice cream, and serve.

Oaty Plum and Apple Crumble

Preparation Time: 20 minutes

Servings 6

Nutrition Values:190 Calories; 7.9g Fat; 28.7g
Carbs; 1.6g Protein; 16.7g Sugars

Ingredients

- 1/4 pound plums, pitted and chopped
- 1/4 pound Braeburn apples, cored and chopped
- 1 tablespoon fresh lemon juice
- 2 ½ ounces golden caster sugar
- 1 tablespoon honey
- 1/2 teaspoon ground mace
- 1/2 teaspoon vanilla paste
- 1 cup fresh cranberries
- 1/3 cup oats
- 2/3 cup flour
- 1/2 stick butter, chilled
- 1 tablespoon cold water

Directions

1. Thoroughly combine the plums and apples with lemon juice, sugar, honey, and ground mace.

2. Spread the fruit mixture onto the bottom of a cake pan that is previously greased with non-stick cooking oil.

3. In a mixing dish, combine the other ingredients until everything is well incorporated. Spread this mixture evenly over the fruit mixture.

4. Air-bake at 390 degrees F for 20 minutes or until done.

Butter Lemon Pound Cake

Preparation Time: 2 hours 20 minutes

Servings 8

Nutrition Values:227 Calories; 9.2g Fat; 34.3g Carbs; 4.2g Protein; 16.6g Sugars

Ingredients

- 1 stick softened butter
- 1/3 cup muscovado sugar
- 1 medium-sized egg
- 1 ¼ cups cake flour
- 1 teaspoon butter flavoring
- 1 teaspoon vanilla essence
- A pinch of salt
- 3/4 cup milk
- Grated zest of 1 medium-sized lemon
- For the Glaze:
- 1 cup powdered sugar
- 2 tablespoons fresh squeezed lemon juice

Directions

1. In a mixing bowl, cream the butter and sugar. Now, fold in the egg and beat again.

2. Add the flour, butter flavoring, vanilla essence, and salt; mix to combine well. Afterward, add the milk and lemon zest and mix on low until everything's incorporated.

3. Evenly spread a thin layer of melted butter all around the cake pan using a pastry brush. Now, press the batter into the cake pan.

4. Bake at 350 degrees F for 15 minutes. After that, take the cake out of the Air Fryer and carefully run a small knife around the edges; invert the cake onto a serving platter. Allow it to cool completely.

5. To make the glaze, mix powdered sugar with lemon juice. Drizzle over the top of your cake and allow hardening for about 2 hours.

Festive Double-Chocolate Cake

Preparation Time: 45 minutes

Servings 8

Nutrition Values:227 Calories; 12.7g Fat; 39.5g Carbs; 3.6g Protein; 24.3g Sugars

Ingredients

- 1/2 cup caster sugar
- 1 ¼ cups cake flour
- 1 teaspoon baking powder
- 1/3 cup cocoa powder
- 1/4 teaspoon ground cloves
- 1/8 teaspoon freshly grated nutmeg
- A pinch of table salt
- 1 egg
- 1/4 cup soda
- 1/4 cup milk
- 1/2 stick butter, melted
- 2 ounces bittersweet chocolate, melted
- 1/2 cup hot water

Directions

1. Take two mixing bowls. Thoroughly combine the dry ingredients in the first bowl. In the second bowl, mix the egg, soda, milk, butter, and chocolate.

2. Add the wet mix to the dry mix; pour in the water and mix well. Butter a cake pan that fits into your Air Fryer. Pour the mixture into the baking pan.

3. Loosely cover with foil; bake at 320 degrees F for 35 minutes. Now, remove foil and bake for further 10 minutes. Frost the cake with buttercream if desired. Bon appétit!

Apple and Pear Crisp with Walnuts

Preparation Time: 25 minutes

Servings 6

Nutrition Values:190 Calories; 5.3g Fat; 33.1g Carbs; 3.6g Protein; 13.7g Sugars

Ingredients

- 1/2 pound apples, cored and chopped
- 1/2 pound pears, cored and chopped
- 1 cup all-purpose flour
- 1/3 cup muscovado sugar
- 1/3 cup brown sugar
- 1 tablespoon butter
- 1 teaspoon ground cinnamon
- 1/4 teaspoon ground cloves
- 1 teaspoon vanilla extract
- 1/4 cup chopped walnuts
- Whipped cream, to serve

Directions

1. Arrange the apples and pears on the bottom of a lightly greased baking dish.

2. Mix the remaining ingredients, without the walnuts and the whipped cream, until the mixture resembles the coarse crumbs.

3. Spread the topping onto the fruits. Scatter chopped walnuts over all.

4. Air-bake at 340 degrees F for 20 minutes or until the topping is golden brown. Check for doneness using a toothpick and serve at room temperature topped with whipped cream.

Family Coconut Banana Treat

Preparation Time: 20 minutes

Servings 6

Nutrition Values:271 Calories; 6.6g Fat; 51.3g Carbs; 4.8g Protein; 19.3g Sugars

Ingredients

- 2 tablespoons coconut oil
- 3/4 cup breadcrumbs
- 2 tablespoons coconut sugar
- 1/2 teaspoon cinnamon powder
- 1/4 teaspoon ground cloves
- 6 ripe bananas, peeled and halved
- 1/3 cup rice flour
- 1 large-sized well-beaten egg

Directions

1. Preheat a non-stick skillet over a moderate heat; stir the coconut oil and the breadcrumbs for about 4 minutes. Remove from the heat, add coconut sugar, cinnamon, and cloves; set it aside.

2. Coat the banana halves with the rice flour, covering on all sides. Then, dip them in beaten egg. Finally, roll them over the crumb mix.

3. Cook in a single layer in the Air Fryer basket at 290 degrees F for 10 minutes. Work in batches as needed.

4. Serve warm or at room temperature sprinkled with flaked coconut if desired. Bon appétit!

Old-Fashioned Swirled German Cake

Preparation Time: 25 minutes

Servings 8

Nutrition Values:278 Calories; 13.1g Fat; 38.7g Carbs; 3.6g Protein; 25.6g Sugars

Ingredients

- 1 cup flour
- 1 teaspoon baking powder
- 1 cup white sugar
- 1/8 teaspoon kosher salt
- 1/4 teaspoon ground cinnamon
- 1/4 teaspoon grated nutmeg
- 1 teaspoon orange zest
- 1 stick butter, melted
- 2 eggs
- 1 teaspoon pure vanilla extract
- 1/4 cup milk
- 2 tablespoons unsweetened cocoa powder

Directions

1. Lightly grease a round pan that fits into your Air Fryer.

2. Combine the flour, baking powder, sugar, salt, cinnamon, nutmeg, and orange zest using an electric mixer. Then, fold in the butter, eggs, vanilla, and milk.

3. Add 1/4 cup of the batter to the baking pan; leave the remaining batter and stir the cocoa into it. Drop by spoonful over the top of white batter. Then, swirl the cocoa batter into the white batter with a knife.

4. Bake at 360 degrees F approximately 15 minutes. Let it cool for about 10 minutes.

5. Finally, turn the cake out onto a wire rack.

Vanilla and Banana Pastry Puffs

Preparation Time: 15 minutes

Servings 8

Nutrition Values:308 Calories; 17.1g Fat; 34.6g Carbs; 5.2g Protein; 18.4g Sugars

Ingredients

- 1 package -8-ouncecrescent dinner rolls, refrigerated
- 1 cup of milk
- 4 ounces instant vanilla pudding
- 4 ounces cream cheese, softened
- 2 bananas, peeled and sliced
- 1 egg, lightly beaten

Directions

1. Unroll crescent dinner rolls; cut into 8 squares.

2. Combine the milk and the pudding; whisk in the cream cheese. Divide the pudding mixture among the pastry squares. Top with the slices of banana.

3. Now, fold the dough over the filling, pressing the edges to help them seal well. Brush each pastry puff with the whisked egg.

4. Air-bake at 355 degrees F for 10 minutes. Bon appétit!

Party Hazelnut Brownie Cups

Preparation Time: 30 minutes

Servings 12

Nutrition Values:246 Calories; 14.5g Fat; 27.5g Carbs; 2.4g Protein; 18.6g Sugars

Ingredients

- 6 ounces semisweet chocolate chips
- 1 stick butter, at room temperature
- 1/2 cup caster sugar
- 1/4 cup brown sugar
- 2 large-sized eggs
- 1/4 cup red wine
- 1/4 teaspoon hazelnut extract
- 1 teaspoon pure vanilla extract
- 3/4 cup all-purpose flour
- 2 tablespoons cocoa powder
- 1/2 cup ground hazelnuts
- A pinch of kosher salt

Directions

1. Microwave the chocolate chips with butter.

2. Then, whisk the sugars, eggs, red wine, hazelnut and vanilla extract. Add to the chocolate mix.

3. Stir in the flour, cocoa powder, ground hazelnuts, and a pinch of kosher salt. Mix until the batter is creamy and smooth. Divide the batter among muffin cups that are coated with cupcake liners.

4. Air-bake at 360 degrees F for 28 to 30 minutes. Bake in batches and serve topped with ganache if desired.

Sultana Cupcakes with Buttercream Icing

Preparation Time: 25 minutes

Servings 6

Nutrition Values:366 Calories; 19.1g Fat; 47.4g Carbs; 2.8g Protein; 38.3g Sugars

Ingredients

For the Cupcakes:

- 1/2 cup all-purpose flour
- 1/2 teaspoon baking soda
- 1 baking powder
- 1/8 teaspoon salt
- 1/4 teaspoon ground anise star
- 1/4 teaspoon grated nutmeg
- 1 teaspoon cinnamon
- 3 tablespoons caster sugar
- 1/2 teaspoon pure vanilla extract
- 1 egg
- 1/4 cup plain milk
- 1/2 stick melted butter

- 1/2 cup Sultanas

For the Buttercream Icing:

- 1/3 cup butter, softened
- 1 ½ cups powdered sugar
- 1 teaspoon vanilla extract
- 1/8 teaspoon salt
- 2 tablespoons milk
- A few drop food coloring

Directions

1. Take two mixing bowls. Thoroughly combine the dry ingredients for the cupcakes into the first bowl. In another bowl, whisk the vanilla extract, egg, milk, and melted butter.

2. To form a batter, add the wet milk mixture to the dry flour mixture. Fold in Sultanas and gently stir to combine. Ladle the batter into the prepared muffin pans.

3. Air-bake at 390 degrees F for 15 minutes.

4. Meanwhile, to make the Buttercream Icing, beat the butter until creamy and fluffy. Gradually add the sugar and beat well.

5. Then, add the vanilla, salt, and milk, and mix until creamy. Afterward, gently stir in food coloring. Frost your cupcakes and enjoy!

Banana & Vanilla Pastry Puffs

Preparation Time: 15 minutes

Smart Points: 4

Servings: 8

Ingredients

- 1 package [8-oz.] crescent dinner rolls, refrigerated
- 1 cup milk
- 4 oz. instant vanilla pudding
- 4 oz. cream cheese, softened
- 2 bananas, peeled and sliced
- 1 egg, lightly beaten

Directions:

1. Roll out the crescent dinner rolls and slice each one into 8 squares.

2. Mix together the milk, pudding, and cream cheese using a whisk.

3. Scoop equal amounts of the mixture into the pastry squares. Add the banana slices on top.

4. Fold the squares around the filling, pressing down on the edges to seal them.

5. Apply a light brushing of the egg to each pastry puff before placing them in the Air Fryer.

6. Air bake at 355°F for 10 minutes.

Double Chocolate Cake

Preparation Time: 45 minutes

Smart Points: 4

Servings: 8

Ingredients

- ½ cup stevia
- 1 ¼ cups keto almond flour
- 1 tsp. baking powder
- ⅓ cup cocoa powder
- ¼ tsp. ground cloves
- 1/8 tsp. freshly grated nutmeg
- Pinch of table salt
- 1 egg
- ¼ cup soda of your choice
- ¼ cup milk
- ½ stick butter, melted
- 2 oz. bittersweet chocolate, melted
- ½ cup hot water

Directions:

1. In a bowl, thoroughly combine the dry ingredients.

2. In another bowl, mix together the egg, soda, milk, butter, and chocolate.

3. Combine the two mixtures. Add in the water and stir well.

4. Take a cake pan that is small enough to fit inside your Air Fryer and transfer the mixture to the pan.

5. Place a sheet of foil on top and bake at 320°F for 35 minutes.

6. Take off the foil and bake for further 10 minutes.

7. Frost the cake with buttercream if desired before serving.

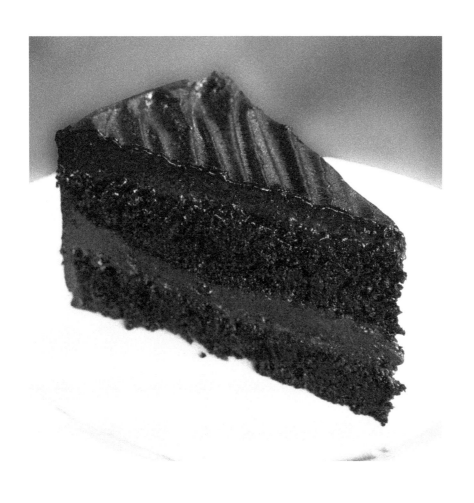

Banana Oatmeal Cookies

Preparation Time: 20 minutes

Smart Points: 3

Servings: 6

Ingredients

- 2 cups quick oats
- ¼ cup milk
- 4 ripe bananas, mashed
- ¼ cup coconut, shredded

Directions:

1. Pre-heat the Air Fryer to 350°F.

2. Combine all of the ingredients in a bowl.

3. Scoop equal amounts of the cookie dough onto a baking sheet and put it in the Air Fryer basket.

4. Bake the cookies for 15 minutes.

Keto Sugar Butter Fritters

Preparation Time: 30 minutes

Smart Points: 4

Servings: 16

Ingredients

For the dough:

- 4 cups keto almond flour
- 1 tsp. kosher salt
- 1 tsp. stevia
- 3 tbsp. butter, at room temperature
- 1 packet instant yeast
- 1 ¼ cups lukewarm water

For the Cakes

- 1 cup stevia
- Pinch of cardamom
- 1 tsp. cinnamon powder
- 1 stick butter, melted

Directions:

1. Place all of the ingredients in a large bowl and combine well.

2. Add in the lukewarm water and mix until a soft, elastic dough forms.

3. Place the dough on a lightly floured surface and lay a greased sheet of aluminum foil on top of the dough. Refrigerate for 5 to 10 minutes.

4. Remove it from the refrigerator and divide it in two. Mold each half into a log and slice it into 20 pieces.

5. In a shallow bowl, combine the stevia, cardamom and cinnamon.

6. Coat the slices with a light brushing of melted butter and the stevia.

7. Spritz Air Fryer basket with cooking spray.

8. Transfer the slices to the fryer and air fry at 360°F for roughly 10 minutes. Turn each slice once during the baking time.

9. Dust each slice with the stevia before serving.

Pear & Apple Crisp with Walnuts

Preparation Time: 25 minutes

Smart Points: 2

Servings: 6

Ingredients

- ½ lb. apples, cored and chopped

- ½ lb. pears, cored and chopped

- 1 cup keto almond flour

- 1 cup stevia

- 1 tbsp. butter

- 1 tsp. ground cinnamon

- ¼ tsp. ground cloves

- 1 tsp. vanilla extract

- ¼ cup chopped walnuts

- Whipped cream, to serve

Directions:

1. Lightly grease a baking dish and place the apples and pears inside.

2. Combine the rest of the ingredients, minus the walnuts and the whipped cream, until a coarse, crumbly texture is achieved.

3. Pour the mixture over the fruits and spread it evenly. Top with the chopped walnuts.

4. Air bake at 340°F for 20 minutes or until the top turns golden brown.

5. When cooked through, serve at room temperature with whipped cream.

Sweet & Crisp Bananas

Preparation Time: 20 minutes

Smart Points: 3

Servings: 4

Ingredients

1. 4 ripe bananas, peeled and halved

2. 1 tbsp. almond meal

3. 1 tbsp. cashew, crushed

4. 1 egg, beaten

5. 1 ½ tbsp. coconut oil

6. ¼ cup keto almond flour

7. 1 ½ tbsp. stevia

8. ½ cup keto friendly bread crumbs

Directions:

1. Put the coconut oil in a saucepan and heat over a medium heat. Stir in the keto bread crumbs and cook, stirring continuously, for 4 minutes.

2. Transfer the keto bread crumbs to a bowl.

3. Add in the almond meal and crushed cashew. Mix well.

4. Coat each of the banana halves in the corn flour, before dipping it in the beaten egg and lastly coating it with the bread crumbs.

5. Put the coated banana halves in the Air Fryer basket. Season with the stevia.

6. Air fry at 350°F for 10 minutes.

Keto Shortbread Fingers

Preparation Time: 20 minutes

Smart Points: 4

Servings: 10

Ingredients

- 1 ½ cups butter
- 1 cup keto almond flour
- ¾ cup stevia
- Cooking spray

Directions:

1. Pre-heat your Air Fryer to 350°F.

2. In a bowl. combine the flour and stevia.

3. Cut each stick of butter into small chunks. Add the chunks into the flour and the stevia.

4. Blend the butter into the mixture to combine everything well.

5. Use your hands to knead the mixture, forming a smooth consistency.

6. Shape the mixture into 10 equal-sized finger shapes, marking them with the tines of a fork for decoration if desired.

7. Lightly spritz the Air Fryer basket with the cooking spray. Place the cookies inside, spacing them out well.

8. Bake the cookies for 12 minutes.

9. Let cool slightly before serving. Alternatively, you can store the cookies in an airtight container for up to 3 days.

Coconut & Banana Cake

Preparation Time: 1 hour 15 minutes

Smart Points: 4

Servings: 5

Ingredients

- 2/3 cup stevia, shaved
- 2/3 cup unsalted butter
- 3 eggs
- 1 ¼ cup keto almond flour
- 1 ripe banana, mashed
- ½ tsp. vanilla extract
- 1/8 tsp. baking soda
- Sea salt to taste

Topping Ingredients

- stevia to taste, shaved
- Walnuts to taste, roughly chopped
- Bananas to taste, sliced

Directions:

1. Pre-heat the Air Fryer to 360°F.

2. Mix together the flour, baking soda, and a pinch of sea salt.

3. In a separate bowl, combine the butter, vanilla extract and stevia using an electrical mixer or a blender, to achieve a fluffy consistency. Beat in the eggs one at a time.

4. Throw in half of the flour mixture and stir thoroughly. Add in the mashed banana and continue to mix. Lastly, throw in the remaining half of the flour mixture and combine until a smooth batter is formed.

5. Transfer the batter to a baking tray and top with the banana slices.

6. Scatter the chopped walnuts on top before dusting with the stevia

7. Place a sheet of foil over the tray and pierce several holes in it.

8. Put the covered tray in the Air Fryer. Cook for 48 minutes.

9. Decrease the temperature to 320°F, take off the foil, and allow to cook for an additional 10 minutes until golden brown.

10.   Insert a skewer or toothpick in the center of the cake. If it comes out clean, the cake is ready.

Roasted Pumpkin Seeds & Cinnamon

Preparation Time: 35 minutes

Smart Points: 3

Servings: 2

Ingredients

- 1 cup pumpkin raw seeds
- 1 tbsp. ground cinnamon
- 2 tbsp. stevia
- 1 cup water
- 1 tbsp. olive oil

Directions:

1. In a frying pan, combine the pumpkin seeds, cinnamon and water.

2. Boil the mixture over a high heat for 2 - 3 minutes.

3. Pour out the water and place the seeds on a clean kitchen towel, allowing them to dry for 20 - 30 minutes.

4. In a bowl, mix together the stevia, dried seeds, a pinch of cinnamon and one tablespoon of olive oil.

5. Pre-heat the Air Fryer to 340°F.

6. Place the seed mixture in the fryer basket and allow to cook for 15 minutes, shaking the basket periodically throughout.

Pineapple Sticks

Preparation Time: 20 minutes

Smart Points:

Servings: 4

Ingredients

- ½ fresh pineapple, cut into sticks
- ¼ cup desiccated coconut

Directions:

1. Pre-heat the Air Fryer to 400°F.

2. Coat the pineapple sticks in the desiccated coconut and put each one in the Air Fryer basket.

3. Air fry for 10 minutes.

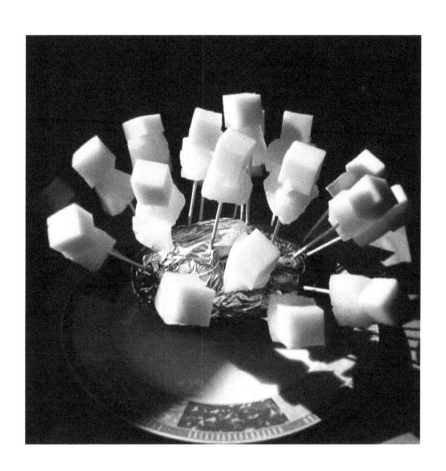

Sponge Cake

Preparation Time: 50 minutes

Smart Points: 5

Servings: 8

Ingredients

For the Cake:

- 9 oz. stevia
- 9 oz. butter
- 3 eggs
- 9 oz. keto almond flour
- 1 tsp. vanilla extract
- Zest of 1 lemon
- 1 tsp. baking powder

For the Frosting

- Juice of 1 lemon
- Zest of 1 lemon
- 1 tsp. yellow food coloring
- 7 oz. stevia
- 4 egg whites

Directions:

1. Pre-heat your Air Fryer to 320°F.

2. Use an electric mixer to combine all of the cake ingredients.

3. Grease the insides of two round cake pans.

4. Pour an equal amount of the batter into each pan.

5. Place one pan in the fryer and cook for 15 minutes, before repeating with the second pan.

6. In the meantime, mix together all of the frosting ingredients.

7. Allow the cakes to cool. Spread the frosting on top of one cake and stack the other cake on top.

Apple Wedges

Preparation Time: 25 minutes

Smart Points: 4

Servings: 4

Ingredients

- 4 large apples
- 2 tbsp. olive oil
- ½ cup dried apricots, chopped
- 1 – 2 tbsp. stevia
- ½ tsp. ground cinnamon

Directions:

1. Peel the apples and slice them into eight wedges. Throw away the cores.

2. Coat the apple wedges with the oil.

3. Place each wedge in the Air Fryer and cook for 12 - 15 minutes at 350°F.

4. Add in the apricots and allow to cook for a further 3 minutes.

5. Stir together the stevia and cinnamon. Sprinkle this mixture over the cooked apples before serving.

Chocolate Lava Cake

Preparation Time: 20 minutes

Smart Points: 3

Servings: 4

Ingredients

- 1 cup dark cocoa candy melts
- 1 stick butter
- 2 eggs
- 4 tbsp. stevia
- 1 tbsp. honey
- 4 tbsp. keto almond flour
- Pinch of kosher salt
- Pinch of ground cloves
- ¼ tsp. grated nutmeg
- ¼ tsp. cinnamon powder

Directions:

1. Spritz the insides of four custard cups with cooking spray.

2. Melt the cocoa candy melts and butter in the microwave for 30 seconds to 1 minute.

3. In a large bowl, combine the eggs, stevia and honey with a whisk until frothy. Pour in the melted chocolate mix.

4. Throw in the rest of the ingredients and combine well with an electric mixer or a manual whisk.

5. Transfer equal portions of the mixture into the prepared custard cups.

6. Place in the Air Fryer and air bake at 350°F for 12 minutes.

7. Remove from the Air Fryer and allow to cool for 5 to 6 minutes.

8. Place each cup upside-down on a dessert plate and let the cake slide out. Serve with fruits and chocolate syrup if desired.

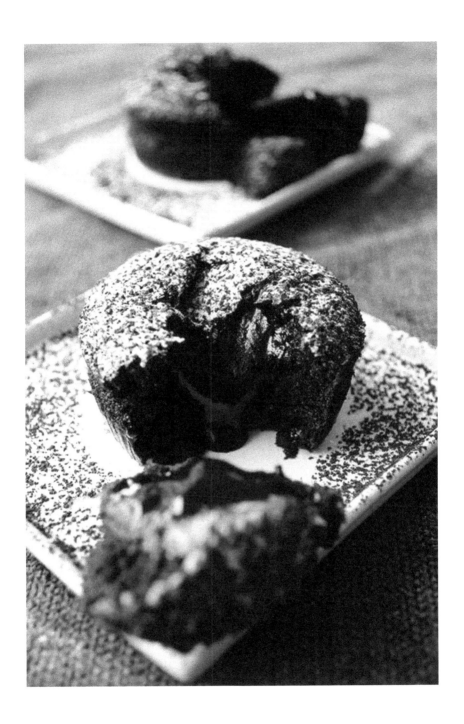

English Lemon Tarts

Preparation Time: 30 minutes

Smart Points: 4

Servings: 4

Ingredients

- ½ cup butter
- ½ lb. keto almond flour
- 2 tbsp. stevia
- 1 large lemon, juiced and zested
- 2 tbsp. lemon curd
- Pinch of nutmeg

Directions:

1. In a large bowl, combine the butter, keto almond flour and stevia until a crumbly consistency is achieved.

2. Add in the lemon zest and juice, followed by a pinch of nutmeg. Continue to combine. If necessary, add a couple tablespoons of water to soften the dough.

3. Sprinkle the insides of a few small pastry tins with flour. Pour equal portions of the

dough into each one and add stevia or lemon zest on top.

4. Pre-heat the Air Fryer to 360°F.

5. Place the lemon tarts inside the fryer and allow to cook for 15 minutes.

Blueberry Pancakes

Preparation Time: 20 minutes

Smart Points: 3

Servings: 4

Ingredients

- ½ tsp. vanilla extract
- 2 tbsp. honey
- ½ cup blueberries
- ½ cup stevia
- 2 cups + 2 tbsp. keto almond flour
- 3 eggs, beaten
- 1 cup milk
- 1 tsp. baking powder
- Pinch of salt

Directions:

1. Pre-heat the Air Fryer to 390°F.

2. In a bowl, mix together all of the dry ingredients.

3. Pour in the wet ingredients and combine with a whisk, ensuring the mixture becomes smooth.

4. Roll each blueberry in some flour to lightly coat it before folding it into the mixture. This is to ensure they do not change the color of the batter.

5. Coat the inside of a baking dish with a little oil or butter.

6. Spoon several equal amounts of the batter onto the baking dish, spreading them into pancake-shapes and ensuring to space them out well. This may have to be completed in two batches.

7. Place the dish in the fryer and bake for about 10 minutes.

New England Pumpkin Cake

Preparation Time: 50 minutes

Smart Points: 3

Servings: 4

Ingredients

- 1 large egg
- ½ cup skimmed milk
- 7 oz. keto almond flour
- 2 tbsp. stevia
- 5 oz. pumpkin puree
- Pinch of salt
- Pinch of cinnamon [if desired]
- Cooking spray

Directions:

1. Stir together the pumpkin puree and stevia in a bowl. Crack in the egg and combine using a whisk until smooth.

2. Add in the flour and salt, stirring constantly. Pour in the milk, ensuring to combine everything well.

3. Spritz a baking tin with cooking spray.

4. Transfer the batter to the baking tin.

5. Pre-heat the Air Fryer to 350°F.

6. Put the tin in the Air Fryer basket and bake for 15 minutes.

Mixed Berry Puffed Pastry

Preparation Time: 20 minutes

Smart Points: 3

Servings: 3

Ingredients

- 3 pastry dough sheets
- ½ cup mixed berries, mashed
- 1 tbsp. honey
- 2 tbsp. cream cheese
- 3 tbsp. chopped walnuts
- ¼ tsp. vanilla extract

Directions:

1. Pre-heat your Air Fryer to 375°F.

2. Roll out the pastry sheets and spread the cream cheese over each one.

3. In a bowl, combine the berries, vanilla extract and honey.

4. Cover a baking sheet with parchment paper.

5. Spoon equal amounts of the berry mixture into the center of each sheet of pastry. Scatter the chopped walnuts on top.

6. Fold up the pastry around the filling and press down the edges with the back of a fork to seal them.

7. Transfer the baking sheet to the Air Fryer and cook for approximately 15 minutes.

Cherry Pie

Preparation Time: 35 minutes

Smart Points: 3

Servings: 8

Ingredients

- 1 tbsp. milk

- 2 ready-made pie crusts

- 21 oz. cherry pie filling

- 1 egg yolk

Directions:

1. Pre-heat the Air Fryer to 310°F.

2. Coat the inside of a pie pan with a little oil or butter and lay one of the pie crusts inside. Use a fork to pierce a few holes in the pastry.

3. Spread the pie filling evenly over the crust.

4. Slice the other crust into strips and place them on top of the pie filling to make the pie look more homemade.

Place in the Air Fryer and cook for 15 minutes.

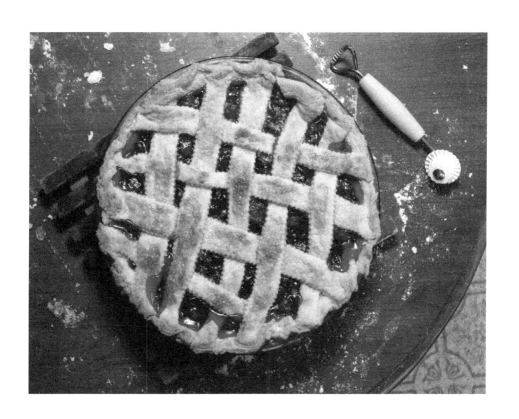

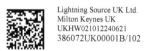

Lightning Source UK Ltd.
Milton Keynes UK
UKHW021012240621
386072UK00001B/102